Low Carb Meal Ideas

Low Carb with Gluten Free and Mediterranean Diet

Kelly Fisher

Table of Contents

Low Carb Meal Ideas

Introduction

Going on a low carb diet has benefits that go beyond simply losing weight. The low carb diet hit a frenzied phase a few years ago, showing many people losing a lot of weight, but also gaining it back as soon as they stopped the diet. The diet came under a lot of scrutiny, being judged as unhealthy, while the proponents held true to their claim of it being perfectly safe and beneficial. This book does not list a "low carb diet" per se but rather features two diets that are naturally low in carbs, but not to the point of being "dangerous." The two diets, the "Gluten Free Diet" and the "Mediterranean Diet" both feature well balanced meals with a lot of fresh fruits and vegetables and good healthy lean meats. Each diet is not strictly "all protein" but offers a nice balance of "good" carbs found in fruits and vegetables along with the protein in lean meats, legumes, and nuts. The diets listed here are modified versions of the famous South Beach and Atkins, without having a "name brand" attached.

The number one "side effect" of a low carb diet is the weight loss, which is why they are so popular with people who need to shed some extra weight and fat. When a low carb diet is consumed the fat and weight fall off faster and easier, and especially with exercise too.

People who suffer from diabetes do well on the low carb diet, because carbs turn into sugar in the body and raises the insulin levels. If a person does not have diabetes, yet it runs in their family they should take measures to prevent it. Eating a low carb diet is a good measure to act as a preventative to the ill health condition.

Reducing the risk for heart disease is another plus of eating a low carb diet. Heart disease is a factor in excessive weight and by losing the weight the risk for heart conditions may go down significantly as well. Preventatives for heart disease are a diet that is high in "good" fats that come from plants like olives. The body needs a healthy balance of good fats and proteins along with "good" carbs derived from fresh fruits and vegetables.

Low carb diets give the body good cholesterol, the kind of cholesterol that works with the body in helping it to be healthier. So as you are losing weight you are gaining good cholesterol. Just an added benefit of these two diet plans.

The Gluten Free diet is primarily a low carb diet because of the absence of gluten. Gluten is found in grains like wheat and in particular, it is found in processed flours and junk foods. Gluten sticks to the body and causes weight gain that turns into fat. Gluten is bad for diabetics because it is a carbohydrate, which the body converts to glucose or sugar. This in turns causes the insulin levels to rise. Even for a non-diabetic, gluten turns into fat. One of the best ways to lose weight is simply to get rid of the gluten, which leaves you with fresh fruits and vegetables and lean cuts of meats. It is easy to shop if you focus on the produce section and the meat counter, and stock up on herbs and spices. However, it is not always easy to come up with different recipes to make the meals go from boring to exciting.

The recipes in the gluten free section of this book can help to plan gluten free meals for two to three weeks or longer. There is a wide variety of meals in the main entree section. For example, try a delicious Turkey Burger. There are Fish Tacos, Gluten Free Lasagna, Seared Ahi Tuna with Grilled Vegetable Quinoa Salad, Gluten Free Beef Stew, Tuscan Style Chicken with Mushrooms, Brazil Nut Crusted Tilapia, Goat Cheese

Ravioli, and Thai Style Peanut Chicken with Gluten Free Noodles.

Appetizers can make great lunches, snacks, or even side dishes. Mix and match these with the main entrees to have a full meal plan. Try the Vinegar Slaw, Balsamic Glazed Roasted Vegetables, Grilled Radicchio with Goat Cheese, Butternut Squash Soup, Sunflower Seed Hummus, or the Gluten Free Pot Stickers.

Breakfast is always an important meal and there are no shortage of recipes and suggestions for the best meal to start the day the low carb way. Breakfast and brunch needs to provide enough food to fuel the body to give energy, get up, and move. Serving these recipes with an additional protein or fruit will be beneficial. Try the Gluten Free Croissants with a slice of lean ham and a piece of fresh fruit. Try the Coconut Flour Pancakes with your favorite low carb toppings. The Crepes go well with fruit too.

The desserts section offers delicious gluten free pies, cookies, and cake. Try the No Bake Strawberry Pie, Brownies with Matcha, Gluten Free Chocolate Chip Cookies or the Pumpkin Cake. There is even a delectable recipe for a Pistachio Cheesecake.

The Mediterranean Diet section contains more suggestions for recipe creation than actual recipes. You will find many of the foods suggestion by the Mediterranean Diet are included in the gluten free recipes. The Mediterranean Diet looks at the people living along the coast of the Mediterranean Sea. These people are healthy, with little heart disease and it is rare to find an obese person. Their diets are rich in the foods produced in their region, fresh fruits and vegetables and very lean cuts of meat. They eat a lot of olive oil in their foods, which provides the body with the good fat and helps the body to combat hypertension, heart disease, and excessive weight gain.

Both of the diets featured below offers low carb diet solutions to help with weight loss and to help develop good eating habits.

Section 1: Gluten Free Weight Loss

What is a Gluten Free Diet? Actually, it makes more sense to answer this question by first addressing what gluten is and why you may want to cut it out of your diet, especially if you're trying to lose weight. Gluten is a protein which is found in most, but not all grains, including wheat, rye, spelt (although to a lesser extent than wheat) and barley.

Gluten derived from grains is also commonly found as an ingredient, additive or binder in a variety of foods, including imitation meat products, condiments, ice cream and other products. For this reason, it's important to check food labels carefully if you're sensitive to gluten or are trying to lose weight through a gluten free diet.

A gluten free diet, as you've probably guessed by now, is a diet which is free of this protein. Although this kind of diet is restrictive in some ways, it definitely doesn't have to be something that makes you feel constantly deprived. As you'll soon find out as you read through and cook the recipes in this book, there are a lot of ways to enjoy the same dishes that you do now while leaving the gluten out.

Gluten Free Diets and Weight Loss Tips

If you've decided to adopt a gluten free diet as part of a larger weight loss program, keep in mind that all of the same rules apply as if you were following any other kind of diet. Regular exercise is an important component of any weight loss regimen and that is no different whether you're cutting gluten out of your life or not.

Additionally, you'll still have to choose what you eat carefully. There are plenty of unhealthy dietary choices out there which are gluten free and it's a mistake to eat just anything because it happens to be gluten free.

This brings us to a statistic which may surprise you. As you may know, many people choose a gluten free diet not necessarily to lose weight, but because they have celiac disease, an intolerance to gluten. According to studies, over 80% of people with gluten sensitivities who switched to a gluten free diet actually gained weight.

Why is this? Because these people didn't follow one of the most basic rules of weight loss – avoiding heavily processed foods. There's a widespread (but false) perception that if a product is labeled as gluten free, it's good for you, but that's not the case. There are many gluten free products on the market which contain nearly twice as many calories as their gluten-containing equivalents.

If you want to lose weight on a gluten free diet, it has to be a healthy diet as well as being free of gluten. This means a diet based on fresh vegetables and fruits, beans, brown rice and other healthy sources of carbohydrates as well as lean proteins. Avoid processed foods where possible and you'll probably find that you don't have a very difficult time losing weight at all.

As long as you follow these basic, common sense weight loss tips, losing weight through eating a healthy gluten free diet and getting regular exercise can be incredibly easy. Since many of the unhealthiest, most heavily processed foods in the typical western diet also contain gluten, cutting out gluten will also mean that you'll be avoiding these dietary pitfalls. Just make sure to replace these unhealthy foods with healthier choices which are also gluten free and you'll be well on your way to weight loss, more energy and better health. Without further delay, let's move on to the recipes.

Entrees

Turkey Tacos

Number of servings: 10 tacos

Ingredients:

10 corn tortillas
1 ½ lbs lean (but not 99% fat free) ground turkey
1 medium sized onion, diced small
3 cloves of garlic, minced
½ cup low sodium chicken broth
½ cup tomato sauce (or mild salsa, if you prefer)
1 tbsp chili powder
1 tsp red wine vinegar
1 tsp oregano
1 tsp vegetable oil

Preparation:

Heat the vegetable oil in a large skillet over medium-high heat. Add the diced onion and cook for about 5 minutes or until mostly softened, stirring regularly. Add the garlic and spices and cook for another minute, stirring occasionally until the garlic becomes fragrant.

Add the ground turkey and cook for about 5 minutes, stirring constantly to break up the meat as it cooks. Cook until cooked through but still just a little bit pink. Add the tomato sauce or salsa, chicken broth, vinegar and bring to a simmer. Cook until thickened and serve hot on warmed corn tortillas with salsa, lime wedges and the condiments, toppings and garnishes of your choice.

Turkey Burgers

Number of servings: 6

Ingredients:

1lb lean ground turkey
1 small red bell pepper, diced small
1 medium sized carrot, diced small
½ of a red onion, diced small
1 small broccoli crown, minced

Preparation:

Add all of the ingredients to a large bowl and mix well to combine. Form into 6 patties and grill until they reach your desired level of doneness. Serve hot on their own or on gluten free buns with the toppings and condiments of your choice.

Thai-Style Peanut Chicken with Gluten Free Noodles

Number of servings: 4

Ingredients:

1 lb cooked chicken breast, cut into bite sized pieces
8 ounces of rice noodles
2 cups snow peas
½ cup spicy Thai style peanut sauce (your choice)
cooking spray

Preparation:

Cook the rice noodles according to the directions on the package and set aside. Cook the snow peas in a skillet lightly coated in cooking spray over medium high heat for about 3 minutes or until cooked through and lightly seared. Add the chicken breast pieces, cooked rice noodles and peanut sauce. Reduce the heat to medium and cook until heated through, stirring regularly to combine the ingredients. Serve hot.

Fish Tacos

Number of servings: 8

Ingredients:

1 lb halibut or tilapia filets, cut into ½" strips
8 corn tortillas
2 cups of coleslaw mix (or shredded cabbage with a little shredded carrot mixed in)
¾ cup mayonnaise
½ packed cup of cilantro, minced
1 jalapeno pepper, minced (remove the seeds for less heat)
2 tbsp rice vinegar or apple cider vinegar
3 tbsp olive oil
3 tsp cumin
3 tsp chili powder, or more to taste
juice of 1 lime
salt and black pepper, to taste
Pico de gallo and lime wedges, for serving

Preparation:

Start by preheating your oven to 325 F. Brush the tortillas with 1 tbsp of the olive oil. Wrap the oiled tortillas in aluminum foil and place in the oven to warm while you prepare the rest of the ingredients.

Add the chopped cilantro, coleslaw mix, minced jalapeno and vinegar to a bowl and mix to combine. Season to taste with salt and black pepper and set aside.

Mix together the mayonnaise, lime juice and the remaining 1 tsp of chili powder and cumin and set aside.

Remove the tortillas from the oven and divide the fish among them. Top each taco with the coleslaw mixture and a drizzle of the spiced mayonnaise. Serve hot with pico de gallo and lime wedges.

Cauliflower Crust Pizza, Hawaiian Style

Number of servings: 3 – 4 (1 12" pizza)

Ingredients:

The crust:
½ of a large cauliflower, shredded (a little more than 2 cups)
1 cup low fat mozzarella cheese, shredded
1 large egg
1 clove of garlic, minced
1 tsp oregano
a dash each of salt and black pepper
The toppings:
½ cup pizza sauce (homemade or premade)
½ cup low fat mozzarella cheese, shredded
3 thick slices of Canadian bacon, sliced into thin strips
½ cup of pineapple chunks (cut into smaller pieces, if desired)

Preparation:

Microwave the shredded cauliflower for 8 minutes in a microwave safe bowl or steam over medium-high heat in a little bit of water until softened; the microwave method is preferable, however. Allow to cool to room temperature.

Preheat your oven to 450 F and spray a pizza pan with cooking spray (or use a non-stick pan). Mix together the cauliflower and the rest of the ingredients for the crust in a bowl. Press the crust mixture into your prepared pizza pan to form a crust and lightly spray with cooking spray. Once the oven is hot, bake the crust for 15 – 17 minutes, or until it turns golden brown. Remove from the oven and increase the heat to broil.

Now you can add the toppings to your crust. Spread the sauce onto the crust, leaving a small border around the edge. Top with half of the shredded mozzarella, Canadian bacon and pineapple pieces, followed by the remainder of the cheese. Broil for 3 – 4 minutes or until the cheese melts, bubbles and browns slightly. Remove from the oven, slice and serve hot.

Sweet Potato and Black Bean Tamales

Number of servings: varies (this recipe will make approximately 20 – 24 tamales)

Ingredients:

50 dried corn husks, soaked overnight plus 3 or 4 extra
1 large poblano pepper, broiled, peeled, seeded and diced small
1 red bell pepper, diced small
1 green bell pepper, diced small
1 sweet potato, diced (may be peeled if desired)
1 can of black beans (15 – 16 ounces), drained and rinsed
1 cup diced tomatoes
½ cup cilantro, chopped
3 green onions, sliced thin
2 cloves of garlic, minced
2 tbsp olive oil
2 tsp cumin
1 tsp oregano

The dough:

2 cups masa dough

4 cups low sodium vegetable broth

2 tsp cumin

2 tsp chili powder

4 tbsp olive oil

1 tsp salt

Preparation:

Take 4 - 5 of the larger corn husks and tear them into ¼"
strips. Place the strips into a bowl of water and set aside.
Preheat your oven to 425 F. Mix together the diced
poblano, sweet potatoes, bell peppers and green onions
in a bowl. Add 1 tbsp olive oil and toss to coat. When the
oven is hot, roast the sweet potato and pepper mixture
on a foil-lined pan for about 25 minutes.

Heat 1 tbsp olive oil in a large heavy skillet over medium
heat. Saute the garlic until browned, then add the
tomatoes, roasted vegetables, black beans, cumin and
cilantro. Remove from heat and set aside while you
prepare the masa dough.

Add the masa flour, olive oil, salt, cumin and chili
powder to a food processor and blend on medium speed
to combine. Reduce the speed to low and add the broth
a little bit at a time until the mixture forms a slightly firm
dough.

Now you're ready to assemble your tamales. Lay two husks on a cutting board or other flat work surface. Place a little dough (slightly less than ¼ of a cup) at the top of two corn husks and flatten it out to cover about 2/3 of the husk, using a plastic bag to prevent the dough from sticking to your fingers. Add about 1 tbsp of the black bean mixture in the center and roll up snugly, then tie closed with one of the soaked corn husk strips. Repeat the procedure until you've used up all of the filling.

Place the tamales in a steamer, standing up with about 2 inches of water. Steam for 1 hour or until the dough easily pulls away from the husk. Serve hot with the salsa of your choice.

Steamed Shrimp and Vegetables

Number of servings: 4

Ingredients:

¾ lb medium sized shrimp, peeled, cleaned and deveined
1 large head of bok choy, sliced about ¼" thin
1 cup snow peas
½ cup shredded carrots
1 clove of garlic, minced
a ½" piece of ginger, peeled and minced or crushed
2 tbsp reduced sodium gluten free soy sauce
1 tbsp toasted sesame oil
1 tsp rice vinegar
1 tsp chili oil
½ tsp brown sugar

Preparation:

Add the garlic, ginger, sesame and chili oil, vinegar, sugar and sesame oil to a small bowl and stir to combine. Place the shrimp in another bowl, add about 1/3 of the liquid and toss to coat. Set aside.

Steam the vegetables and shrimp until the shrimp is just cooked through, about 10 minutes. Remove from heat, toss with the rest of the sauce and serve hot over steamed brown rice and chili paste on the side.

Gluten Free Lasagna

Number of servings: 6 - 8

Ingredients:

2 (10 ounce) boxes gluten free lasagna noodles
2 lbs lean ground beef
3 ½ cups marinara sauce (store bought or homemade)
2 cups ricotta cheese
2 cups low fat mozzarella cheese, shredded
½ cup grated Parmesan or Romano cheese
½ cup fresh basil, finely chopped
½ cup Italian parsley, finely chopped
1 large red onion, diced small
4 cloves of garlic, minced (or more to taste)
2 eggs, lightly beaten
4 tbsp olive oil
2 tbsp Italian seasoning
1 tbsp fennel seeds, coarsely ground
2 tsp salt

Preparation:

Preheat your oven to 350 F while you get everything
ready. Bring a large stockpot 2/3 filled with cold water to

a rolling boil. Add 1 tbsp olive oil and 1 tsp salt, add 14 of the noodles and boil until al dente, about 12 – 13 minutes. Drain the noodles and rinse with cold water. Toss with 1 tbsp olive oil to prevent from sticking together and set aside.

In a large skillet, sauté the garlic and onion in 3 tbsp olive oil for 2 minutes, stirring occasionally. Add the ground beef and 1 tsp salt and cook until browned, stirring occasionally. Add the marinara sauce, half of the Italian seasoning and the fennel seeds. Stir and cook for 10 minutes, stirring as needed to keep the mixture from burning. Remove from heat and set aside.

Mix together the ricotta and Parmesan or Romano, the eggs, basil, parsley, oregano and black pepper to taste in a medium sized bowl and set aside. Now you're ready to put it all together. Spread the bottom of a 9" baking dish with the meat sauce, then a layer of lasagna noodles (it should take 4 noodles, overlapped to do this).

Follow this with a layer of the cheese mixture and a sprinkling of mozzarella. Repeat until you've used up all of the noodles, then top with the remaining sauce, mozzarella and the other 1 tbsp of Italian seasoning. Bake for about 1 hour, or until the top is golden brown. Remove from heat and allow the lasagna to rest for at least ten minutes, then slice and serve.

Butternut Squash Risotto

Number of servings: 4 – 6

Ingredients:

1 small butternut squash, peeled, seeded and diced
1 cup Arborio rice
4 cups vegetable broth, warmed
¼ cup dry sherry (not cooking sherry)
2 shallots, minced
2 cloves of garlic, minced
2 tbsp unsalted butter
2 tbsp olive oil
salt, black pepper and chopped fresh sage, to taste

Preparation:

Heat the olive oil and butter in a large saucepan over medium heat. Once the oil and butter are hot, add the shallots and a little black pepper and sauté until softened, about 3 minutes. Add the garlic and a pinch of salt, stir and cook for another minute. Add the cubed squash and cook for about 10 minutes or until the squash starts to soften, about 10 minutes. Add the rice and cook for another 1 – 2 minutes, stirring regularly to prevent burning.

Add the sherry and cook until the alcohol cooks off and the rice absorbs the remaining liquid. Add ½ cup of vegetable broth and continue to cook at a simmer, stirring constantly until the broth is absorbed. Repeat until the broth is all absorbed and the rice is tender and takes on a creamy texture, 15 – 20 minutes. Sprinkle with chopped sage and serve hot.

Seared Ahi Tuna with Grilled Vegetable Quinoa Salad

Number of servings: 8

Ingredients:

2 lbs ahi tuna
2 cups dry quinoa
2 zucchini, sliced lengthwise
2 yellow summer squash, sliced lengthwise
2 small eggplants, sliced lengthwise
2 large Portabella mushrooms, sliced
1 large yellow or white onion, sliced
4 Roma tomatoes, diced
4 ½ cups low sodium vegetable stock
4 tbsp olive oil
2 tbsp rice vinegar or apple cider vinegar
2 tsp dried chives (or 2 tbsp fresh chives, if available)
2 tsp tarragon
2 tsp thyme
salt and black pepper, to taste
1 head of raddichio, for serving
cooking spray

Preparation:

Rinse the quinoa well in a strainer while you bring the vegetable stock to a boil in a medium saucepan. Add the quinoa and thyme, reduce heat, cover and simmer until the quinoa absorbs the liquid and becomes fluffy, about 15 minutes. Fluff the quinoa with a fork and set aside.

Spray a skillet with cooking spray and cook the vegetables over medium heat until they're tender. Remove from heat and set aside. After giving the vegetables a few minutes to cool, dice them into small pieces. Add the diced vegetables, quinoa, tomatoes and remaining herbs to a bowl and toss to mix. Add black pepper to taste, stir again and set aside.

Season the tuna with black pepper and brush with 1 tbsp olive oil while you heat a nonstick skillet over high heat. Sear the tuna on each side and remove from heat. Transfer the tuna to a cutting board and cut into thin slices with a sharp knife. Arrange radicchio leaves on serving plates, topped with quinoa salad and a portion of the tuna slices. Serve immediately.

Blackened Shrimp Nachos

Number of servings: 4

Ingredients:

½ lb cooked shrimp, tails removed
½ of a red bell pepper, diced small
½ cup shredded Monterey Jack or cheddar cheese
1 small jalapeno, sliced thinly
2 tbsp chopped cilantro
2 tbsp Italian dressing
gluten-free tortilla chips
1 tsp sweet (Hungarian) paprika
2 tsp salt
1 tsp black pepper
1 tsp garlic powder
½ tsp cayenne pepper, or more to taste
salsa, for serving

Preparation:

Preheat your oven to 375 F. Heat a large, non-stick
skillet over high heat until very hot. Add ½ of the Italian
dressing, the diced bell peppers and the spices. Cook for
about 1 – 1 ½ minutes or until the pepper begins to look

roasted, stirring regularly. Add the shrimp and cook, stirring regularly until the shrimp is well coated with the spice mixture and cooked through. Add the remaining dressing, remove from heat and set aside.

Arrange tortilla chips in a single layer on a baking sheet, topped with half of the shrimp and cheese. Add a second layer of tortilla chips, then the remaining shrimp and cheese, then top with the sliced jalapenos. Bake for about 10 minutes, or until the cheese is melted and slightly browned. Remove from heat and top with chopped cilantro. Serve at once with the salsa of your choice.

Gluten-Free Beef Stew

Number of servings: 6 - 8

Ingredients:

1 lb lean beef stew meat
1 lb red potatoes, cubed
2 cups diced tomatoes
2 cups beef stock
1 cup fresh or frozen peas
1 cup fresh or frozen corn
1 medium sized yellow onion, diced
3 medium sized carrots, sliced
3 cloves of garlic, sliced
2 tbsp brandy (optional)
2 tbsp rice flour
2 tbsp potato starch
1 tbsp olive oil
1 tsp each thyme and oregano
salt and black pepper, to taste

Preparation:

Mix together the rice flour, potato starch, salt, pepper
and herbs in a large bowl with a lid. Add the beef, close

and shake well to coat. Heat the olive oil in a large skillet over medium high heat. Place the beef in the skillet (save the remaining flour mixture for later) and cook for about 3 minutes per side or until just browned. Add the brandy (if using) and cook for another minute. Remove from heat and set aside.

Add the beef stock, onions, carrots and tomatoes to a large saucepan or stock pot over medium heat. Add 1 tbsp of the remaining flour mixture and stir to coat. Add the beef, reduce to a simmer and cook, covered for 2 hours. Add the potatoes and cook for another 30 – 35 minutes or until the potatoes are tender. Add the corn and peas and cook for 10 – 15 minutes or until heated through. Season to taste with salt and black pepper and serve hot.

Orange Chicken

Number of servings: 4

Ingredients:

2 skinless, boneless chicken breasts, cut into bite sized pieces
2 cups cooked brown rice, kept warm

3 cups shredded Savoy cabbage or green cabbage

1 red bell pepper, sliced into strips

1 cup small broccoli florets

4 green onions, trimmed and sliced thinly

1 cup San-J brand orange sauce

¼ cup corn starch

2 tbsp canola oil

chili sauce, to taste

Preparation:

Toss the chicken and corn starch in a bowl or bag to coat while you heat the oil in a large skillet or wok over medium heat. Add the chicken pieces and cook, stirring occasionally until the chicken is cooked through and slightly crisp on the outside; this will take 5 minutes or less. Remove the chicken and set aside.

Add the vegetables to the skillet and cook for about 5 minutes or until slightly reduced and heated through, stirring regularly. Return the chicken to the pan along with the orange sauce and a little chili sauce. Stir and continue cooking for another 1 - 2 minutes or until heated through. Serve hot over brown rice.

Tuna Casserole

Number of servings: 4

Ingredients:

8 ounces gluten free pasta (your choice, but small shells work the best)
1 12 ounce can of tuna in water, drained and broken up into small pieces
1 small yellow onion, diced
½ of a red bell pepper, diced small
1 cup frozen or fresh peas
1 cup shredded sharp cheddar cheese
1 cup gluten free bread or cracker crumbs
1 cup gluten free cream of mushroom soup
1 ½ cups milk
4 tbsp rice flour
2 tbsp butter
1 tbsp olive oil
salt and black pepper, to taste

Preparation:

Preheat your oven to 350 F. Cook the pasta according to the directions on the package. Just before the pasta is done, add the peas. Drain and rinse in cold water, then pour into a large bowl and set aside.

Melt the butter in a saucepan over medium heat, then add the onion and bell pepper and sauté for about 3 minutes, stirring occasionally. Add the rice flour, stir to combine and continue to cook for another 3 minutes, stirring regularly. Add the mushroom soup, milk and salt and pepper to taste. Whisk to combine. Reduce to a simmer and continue stirring until the mixture thickens.

Pour the thickened sauce over the pasta and peas, followed by the tuna and half of the cheese. Stir to combine. Pour the mixture into a 9" x 13" baking dish and top with the other half of the cheese. Mix together the bread or cracker crumbs and olive oil until combined and sprinkle over the casserole. Bake for 40 minutes or until the casserole is bubbling and nicely browned. Remove from the oven and allow to rest for 5 minutes before serving.

Goat Cheese Ravioli

Number of servings: 4

Ingredients:

8 gluten free lasagna sheets
1 large (28 ounce) can of whole tomatoes with juice
2 tbsp unsalted butter
2 tbsp minced shallots
1 tbsp olive oil
1 tsp Italian seasoning
salt, black pepper and red pepper flakes, to taste
The filling:
1 cup goat cheese
¼ cup arugula leaves, chopped
1 clove of garlic, minced or crushed
2 tbsp olive oil
1 tsp lemon zest
1 tsp black pepper
salt and black pepper, to taste

Preparation:

Cook the pasta according to the directions on the package, drain and rinse in cold water. Transfer the cooked pasta to a cutting board and slice each noodle into 3 pieces. Place between damp towels and set aside.

Next, make your sauce. Heat 1 tbsp of olive oil in a medium sized saucepan over medium heat. Saute the shallots, red pepper flakes (if desired) and Italian seasoning until the shallots turn transparent, stirring occasionally. Add the tomatoes, reduce the heat to low and simmer for 30 minutes, stirring regularly until the tomatoes break down and form a sauce. Add the butter and continue simmering until it melts, stirring to combine. Season to taste with salt and black pepper, remove from heat and cover to keep warm.

Preheat your oven to 375 F and start making the filling. Saute the garlic in the other tbsp of olive oil over medium heat until golden brown, 2 – 3 minutes. Add the arugula, lemon zest and black pepper and cook for about 2 minutes or until the arugula is wilted, stirring frequently. Transfer the arugula to a cutting board, allow to cool for a few minutes, chop finely and transfer to a bowl along with the goat cheese. Stir to combine and set aside.

Spray a 9" x 13" baking dish with cooking spray and place half of the pasta squares in the dish. Top each square with about 1 tbs of the filling and cover with another pasta square. Pour the sauce over the ravioli and bake for about 15 minutes, or until heated through. Remove from the oven and serve at once.

Shrimp and Tofu Pad Thai

Number of servings: 4

Ingredients:

½ lb medium sized shrimp, cleaned, peeled and deveined (if frozen, thaw first)
8 oz rice noodles
8 oz firm tofu, cubed
3 tbsp vegetable oil
2 eggs, lightly beaten
1 small onion, thinly sliced
2 cloves of garlic, minced
1 cup shredded carrots
1 cup gluten free Pad Thai sauce (your choice)
2 tbsp chopped cilantro, 2 tbsp chopped roasted peanuts, green onion slices and lime wedges, for garnish

Preparation:

Cook the rice noodles as per the directions on the package. Rinse with cold water in a colander and set aside. Heat 1 tbsp of the vegetable oil in a large skillet or wok over high heat. Add the eggs and scramble, stirring constantly to prevent burning. Remove from the skillet or wok, place in a bowl and set aside.

Add the rest of the vegetable oil to the skillet or wok and heat. Add the shrimp and onion and cook, stirring frequently, until the shrimp are cooked through and opaque. Add the garlic and ginger and cook for another minute, then transfer to the bowl along with the eggs and reduce the heat to low. Return the noodles to the skillet or wok along with the Pad Thai sauce and stir to combine. Return the shrimp, eggs, followed by the rest of the ingredients. Serve immediately, garnished with the peanuts, cilantro, green onions and lime wedges.

Tuna Melt Tostadas

Number of servings: 2

Ingredients:

1/3 cup tuna in water, drained
2 corn tortillas
1 tsp mayonnaise
1 tsp pickle relish or diced dill pickle
½ tsp brown mustard
4 tbsp shredded cheddar cheese
cooking spray

Preparation:

Start by preheating your oven to 400 F. Mix together the tuna, mustard, mayonnaise and relish or diced pickle in a bowl. Set aside. Lightly coat a baking sheet with cooking spray and place the tortillas on the prepared baking sheet. Lightly spray the tops of the tortillas and bake until they begin to brown and become crisp. Remove from the oven, top with the tuna mixture and shredded cheddar cheese. Return to the oven and bake until the cheese is melted to your liking. Remove from the oven and serve immediately.

Mussels over Pasta

Number of servings: 4

Ingredients:

2 lbs live mussels, scrubbed well and rinsed
8 ounces gluten free linguini or fettucine, cooked
1 small celery stalk, diced
½ of a small white or yellow onion, diced
2 cloves of garlic, minced
juice of ½ lemon
1 cup water
2 tbsp Italian parsley, chopped
2 tbsp fresh basil, chopped
2 tbsp olive oil (use extra virgin olive oil for this recipe, if you have it on hand)
salt and black pepper, to taste

Preparation:

First, make sure that your mussels are still alive. Tap them lightly against the side of your sink; they should make a dull sound, not a hollow sound – they'll also close their shells if they're alive. Scrub the mussels well, taking care to remove their bears and rinse well. Set aside.

In a large saucepan, sauté the garlic and onion in olive oil over medium heat until the garlic turns golden brown. Add the celery, parsley, water, lemon juice and a little salt and pepper and bring the mixture to a boil. Add the basil and mussels, cover and steam for 5 – 10 minutes, or until all of the mussels have opened. Remove from heat and discard any unopened mussels. Serve in bowls over a portion of the cooked pasta.

Pork Chops With Mushroom – Pomegranate Sauce

Number of servings: 4

Ingredients:

1 lb pork (or lamb) chops rubbed with 1 tsp thyme
1 cup button or crimini mushrooms, sliced
½ of a medium-sized yellow onion, minced
3 cloves of garlic, minced
2 tbsp olive oil
salt and black pepper, to taste

The sauce:

1 cup of pomegranate juice
1 tbsp rice vinegar
1 tbsp corn starch
½ tablespoon honey

Preparation:

Preheat your oven to 350 F. Heat the olive oil a large, heavy skillet (a cast iron skillet works well) over medium-high heat and sauté the mushrooms, onions and garlic until tender. Transfer to a bowl and set aside. Add the pork chops to the skillet and cook for 6 minutes per side, then remove from the pan. Whisk together the ingredients for the pomegranate sauce and pour into the pan. Deglaze the pan briefly and return the pork to the skillet.

Return the mushroom mixture to the skillet and transfer to the oven to cook for another 10 – 15 minutes, or until the pork chops are cooked through and the sauce is thickened. Remove from the oven and serve hot over brown rice or gluten free pasta.

Stuffed Potatoes

Number of servings: 2

Ingredients:

2 large russet potatoes, washed and pierced with a fork
2 hardboiled eggs, mashed
4 tbsp shredded Manchego cheese
2 tbsp diced tomato
black pepper, to taste
The tuna salad:
1/2 cup tuna in water, drained
2 tbsp mayonnaise
1 tbsp diced celery
1 tbsp green onion slices
1 tsp Dijon mustard
salt and black pepper, to taste

Preparation:

Bake or microwave the potatoes. While they're cooking, combine the ingredients for the tuna salad and refrigerate until you're ready to use it. Slice the potatoes lengthwise and use a fork to mash the insides. Stir in the cheese, followed by the tuna salad, then the mashed egg and finally the diced tomato. Season to taste with black pepper and serve immediately.

Tuscan Style Chicken with Mushrooms

Number of servings: 4

Ingredients:

1 whole fryer chicken (3 – 3 ½ lbs), disjointed
2 cups cooked gluten free pasta (your choice)
¾ cup sliced crimini mushrooms
¾ cup diced carrots
¾ cup water
½ cup diced celery
¼ cup olive oil
3 tbsp chopped Italian parsley
2 cloves of garlic, chopped
1 medium sized tomato, diced
1 tbsp red wine vinegar
½ tsp basil
½ tsp salt
½ tsp black pepper, or more to taste

Preparation:

Heat the olive oil in a large skillet over medium heat; once the oil is hot, add the chicken and fry until browned on both sides. Move the chicken over to the side of the pan and add the mushrooms. Cook until the mushrooms release their water and turn slightly golden, about 3 minutes. Add the celery, garlic and carrots and cook for another 3 minutes, stirring regularly. Add the salt, pepper, basil, vinegar, tomato and parsley and cook for 3 more minutes, stirring occasionally. Add the water, reduce the heat to low and cover. Cook, covered for 25 minutes. Remove the chicken and transfer to serving plates. Add the pasta to the skillet and stir to combine with the vegetables. Cook for 1 -2 minutes or until the pasta is heated through. Serve immediately.

Stuffed Cabbage

Number of servings: 4 - 6 (2 -3 cabbage leaves per serving)

Ingredients:

1 lb lean ground turkey
12 large green cabbage leaves
1 cup white or parboiled brown rice, uncooked
½ tsp salt
¼ black pepper, or more to taste
The sauce:
4 cups tomato sauce (your choice or homemade)
4 cups of reserved water from cooking the cabbage
½ tsp cinnamon
½ tsp salt

Preparation:

Core a head of cabbage and soak in a large bowl (or clean sink) full of hot water for 10 minutes. Remove and carefully peel off 12 cabbage leaves or a few extra in case you end up tearing one while stuffing them. Bring 6 cups of water to a boil in a large pot and add the cabbage leaves. Cook for a few minutes to blanch and soften, but not thoroughly cook the leaves. Remove and transfer to a plate. Reserve 4 cups of the cooking water and discard the rest.

Mix together the ground turkey in a bowl with the rice, salt and pepper. Add about ¼ cup of the turkey mixture to the inside of each leaf and roll up, burrito style, to close. Repeat the process until you've used up all of the filling.

Add the tomato sauce to the pot with the reserved cooking water and lay your extra cabbage leaves on the bottom to prevent the rolls from sticking to the pot. Arrange the cabbage rolls in the pot, bring to a boil and then reduce the heat to a low simmer and cook for 35 – 40 minutes. Remove the rolls carefully and serve hot.

Brazil Nut-Crusted Tilapia

Number of servings: 3

Ingredients:

3 tilapia filets (4 – 6 ounces each)
1 cup brazil nuts, chopped
3 tbsp crushed gluten free corn flakes
3 tbsp olive oil
3 tbsp milk
salt and black pepper, to taste

Preparation:

Start by preheating your oven to 350 F. Mix together the brazil nuts, crushed corn flakes and some salt and pepper on a large plate. Pour the milk onto another plate. Dip the filets in milk, then roll in the brazil nut mixture until thickly coated. Spread the olive oil on a baking sheet and add the filets. Bake for about 20 minutes or until the fish flakes easily with a fork. Remove from the oven and serve at once.

Appetizers, Side Dishes and Soups

Cucumber - Chickpea Bruschetta

Number of servings: varies

Ingredients:

1 large or 2 small cucumbers, sliced about ¼" – 1/3" thick
1 can of chickpeas, drained, rinsed and mashed
juice of ½ lemon
finely diced tomatoes and red onions, chopped dill and black pepper, for garnish
salt and black pepper, to taste

Preparation:

Mix the mashed chickpeas with lemon juice and a little salt and black pepper, stirring well to combine. Spread the cucumber slices with the chickpeas, transfer to a serving plate and set aside. In a bowl, mix together the tomatoes, onion, herbs and salt and black pepper to taste. Add a small spoonful of the mixture to each cucumber slice and serve immediately or refrigerate for a few hours and serve chilled.

Vinegar Slaw

Number of servings: varies

Ingredients:

2 cups shredded cabbage (green, red or Savoy, your choice)
½ cup shredded carrot
2 tbsp honey
2 tbsp apple cider vinegar, or more to taste
2 tbsp water
salt and black pepper, to taste

Preparation:

Nothing could be easier than preparing this recipe. Simply add all of the ingredients to a large bowl, stir or toss well to combine. Serve at once or refrigerate for a few hours or overnight to allow the flavors to blend.

Balsamic Glazed Roasted Vegetables

Number of servings: 4

Ingredients:

10 large Brussels sprouts, trimmed and halved
4 large carrots, quartered and cut into 2" slices
3 cloves of garlic, minced
1 large shallot, minced
½ cup balsamic vinegar
2 tbsp butter
2 sprigs of fresh thyme or 1 tsp dried thyme

Preparation:

Preheat your oven to 400 F. Melt the butter in a small saucepan over medium – high heat. Add the garlic and shallots and sauté for about 3 minutes or until the garlic starts to become tender. Add the thyme and cook for another minute, stirring occasionally. Add the vinegar and allow the mixture to reduce for about 3 minutes. Allow the sauce to rest for a few minutes, then toss in a large bowl with the vegetables.

Line a baking sheet with foil and spread out the

vegetables on the sheet. Bake for 25 minutes, remove from the oven and serve hot.

Quinoa Ranch Salad

Number of servings: 6

Ingredients:

2 cups water
1 red bell pepper, diced
1 yellow bell pepper, diced
4 green onions, trimmed and sliced thinly
1 ½ cups cooked black beans (drain and rinse if using canned beans)
1 cup quinoa, uncooked
1 cup finely diced sweet potato
1 cup gluten free ranch dressing (your choice or homemade)
½ cup pepitas
¼ cup Italian parsley, chopped
salt and black pepper, to taste

Preparation:

Rinse the quinoa well in a colander, place in a medium saucepan and add the water. Bring to a boil briefly, reduce the heat to simmer and cook, covered for about 12 minutes or until the quinoa has absorbed almost all of the water. Remove from heat but keep covered and allow to rest for 10 minutes before removing the lid and placing into your freezer to cool.

Place the remaining ingredients in a large bowl, add the quinoa and sweet potato once cooled and mix well. Pour the ranch dressing over the salad and stir well to coat. Serve at once or refrigerate, covered and serve chilled.

Sunflower Seed Hummus

Number of servings: varies

Ingredients:

2 (15 ounce) cans of chickpeas, drained and rinsed well
1 cup unsalted sunflower seeds (roasted or raw, your choice)
6 cloves of garlic
1 ½ tbsp olive oil (use extra virgin olive oil for this recipe)
2 tbsp water
juice of 1 lemon or more to taste
salt and black pepper, to taste
a pinch of paprika

Preparation:

Add the garlic and sunflower seeds to a food processor and pulse until they reach the consistency of a coarse meal. Add the remaining ingredients and process until it reaches the consistency you like. Add a little extra water or lemon juice if needed. Season to taste with salt and black pepper, transfer to a serving bowl and sprinkle with paprika and sunflower seeds. Serve at once or refrigerate, covered and serve chilled.

Zucchini and Leek Soup

Number of servings: 6 - 8

Ingredients:

5 leeks, green parts removed, sliced and thoroughly cleaned
6 cups sliced zucchini or yellow summer squash
4 cups of low sodium vegetable or chicken stock
4 cloves of garlic, minced
½ cup coconut milk
½ cup dry white wine
3 tbsp olive oil
1 tbsp apple cider vinegar
1 tbsp dill
salt and black pepper, to taste

Preparation:

Heat a very large saucepan or stock pot over medium heat for 30 seconds to one minute. Add the olive oil and continue to heat for 1 minute. Add the zucchini, leeks and garlic and cook for about 5 minutes, stirring occasionally.

Add the wine and vegetable or chicken stock and bring the soup to a boil. Reduce the heat to a simmer and cook, covered for 30 minutes. Add the vinegar, coconut milk, dill and a little salt and pepper and heat through. Transfer the soup to a blender in batches (or use a hand blender) and blend until smooth and creamy. Season to taste with salt and black pepper and serve hot.

Cranberry Glazed Carrots

Number of servings: 6

Ingredients:

2 lbs baby carrots
½ cup cranberry sauce (whole berry or jellied, your choice)
2 tbsp butter
2 tbsp brown sugar
1 tbsp lemon juice
salt and black pepper, to taste

Preparation:

Add the carrots to a large saucepan with about 1" of water. Bring to a boil, then reduce the heat and simmer, covered for 10 minutes, or until the carrots are tender. Drain and transfer to a bowl. Add the remaining ingredients to the pan and cook over medium heat, stirring regularly, until the mixture is smooth. Return the carrots to the pan, stir well to coat and continue cooking until the carrots are heated through. Serve at once.

Grilled Radicchio with Goat Cheese

Number of servings: 8

Ingredients:

2 heads of radicchio
2 cloves of garlic, minced
½ cup olive oil (use extra virgin olive oil, if you have it on hand)
½ cup goat cheese
¼ cup balsamic vinegar
2 tbsp chopped basil
salt and black pepper, to taste

Preparation:

Quarter the radicchio (don't remove the stem end) and soak in ice water for 1 hour. Meanwhile, whisk together the garlic, vinegar and olive oil in a bowl and set aside. Start your grill, drain the radicchio and place on paper towels to soak up excess water. Open up each quarter, spoon in a portion of the dressing and season with a little salt and pepper.

Once the grill is ready, cook the radicchio for about 3

minutes per side. Remove from the grill and stuff with goat cheese and chopped basil. If there's any of the dressing left, spoon it on top before serving.

Tex-Mex Style Summer Squash

Number of servings: 4

Ingredients:

2 cups cubed yellow summer squash or zucchini
1 cup cooked brown rice, cooled to room temperature
½ cup refried black beans
1/3 cup water
1 tbsp chopped cilantro
1 tsp cumin
salt and black pepper, to taste
salsa, for serving (your choice)

Preparation:

Bring the water to a boil in a medium sized saucepan. Add the squash and a little salt and black pepper. Reduce to a simmer and cook for 5 minutes or until the squash is just beginning to become tender. Add the rice, cumin, refried beans and chopped cilantro. Cook for another 2 – 3 minutes to heat through, stirring occasionally. Serve hot with the salsa of your choice.

Butternut Squash Soup

Number of servings: 4 - 6

Ingredients:

1 large butternut squash (about 2 lbs)
2 cups of low sodium chicken or vegetable stock
1 cup of diced yellow onion
½ cup thinly sliced carrots
¼ cup heavy cream
2 cloves of garlic, chopped
½ of a jalapeno pepper, minced
2 tablespoons peanut oil
1 tsp cumin
salt and black pepper, to taste

Preparation:

Halve the squash lengthwise and remove the seeds and surrounding pulp. Peel the squash and cut into 1" cubes. Heat the peanut oil in a large saucepan or stock pot over medium heat. Once the oil is hot, add the garlic and onion and cook until they start to brown, stirring frequently (about 5 minutes). Add the carrots, cumin and a little salt and pepper and cook for another minute, stirring occasionally.

Add the jalapeno, squash and chicken or vegetable stock and bring to a boil. Reduce the heat and simmer, covered, for 20 minutes or until the squash is tender. Remove from heat and puree in batches in a blender or use a hand blender to blend the soup until smooth. Return the soup to the pot over medium heat, whisk in the cream and season to taste with salt and black pepper. Remove from heat and serve hot.

Gluten-free Pot Stickers

Number of servings: 6 (about 24 pot stickers)

Ingredients:

The wrappers:
1 cup brown rice flour
2/3 cup boiling water
½ cup tapioca flour
¼ cup white rice flour
2 tbsp canola oil
½ tsp salt
¼ tsp xanthan gum
cornstarch, for rolling
The filling:
1 lb lean ground pork
2 green onions, trimmed and sliced thinly
2 cloves of garlic, minced
1 tsp fresh ginger, minced or crushed
1 tbsp sesame oil
salt and black pepper, to taste

Preparation:

Add all of the ingredients to a large bowl and mix well to

combine. Set aside. Mix together the dry ingredients for the wrappers and add boiling water a little bit at a time, mixing with a chopstick. Once the dough is cool enough to handle, knead gently with your hands until the dough reaches the consistency of modeling clay (think Play-Doh). Roll the dough into a log and cut in half. Place one half in a plastic bag until you're ready to use it.

Cut the other half of the dough into 12 pieces and roll each piece into a flat circle of dough. Sprinkle each with corn starch and roll out in between two sheets of plastic wrap until very thin. Roll out 6 wrappers at a time. Brush a wrapper with a little water and add 2 tsp of the filling to the middle, fold over and seal. Set aside. Repeat the process until you've made all 24 pot stickers.

Heat the oil in a large skillet over medium heat, add as many pot stickers as will fit and cook for 2 minutes or until slightly browned. Add ¼ cup water and cook, covered for 8 minutes. Remove the cover and cook uncovered for 3 more minutes or until well browned. Repeat until you've cooked all of the pot stickers and serve hot with the condiments of your choice.

Creamy Cauliflower Soup

Number of servings: 2

Ingredients:

1 ½ fresh or frozen cauliflower florets
1 cup of low sodium chicken or vegetable broth
3 wedges of Laughing Cow (or other brand) light cheese
with garlic and herbs
2 tbsp low fat cheddar cheese
1 tbsp chopped chives
1 tbsp cooked, crumbled turkey bacon
salt and black pepper, to taste

Preparation:

Bring the cauliflower and vegetable or chicken broth to a
boil in a medium saucepan. Reduce to a simmer and
cook, covered for about 15 minutes, or until the
cauliflower starts to fall apart (the cooking time will be
less if you're using frozen cauliflower). Remove from
heat and add to a blender with the garlic and herb
cheese and a little salt and black pepper. Blend until
smooth and transfer to a bowl. Stir in the chives and
cheddar cheese, divide among 2 bowls and top each

with half of the crumbled turkey bacon. Serve
immediately.

Prosciutto Wrapped Basil Shrimp

Number of servings: 4 (5 shrimp per serving)

Ingredients:

20 large shrimp, peeled, deveined and cleaned (and thawed, if frozen)
10 very thinly sliced pieces of prosciutto
1 tbsp of chopped basil
1 tsp olive oil (use extra virgin olive oil for this recipe if you have some on hand)
1 tsp lemon zest
½ tsp salt
½ tsp crushed red pepper flakes
a pinch of black pepper
cooking spray
lemon wedges, for serving

Preparation:

Start by preheating your oven to broil. Add the shrimp, olive oil, chopped basil, lemon zest, salt, black pepper and red pepper flakes. Toss to coat the shrimp with the other ingredients and set aside until later.

Lay out the slices of prosciutto on a large, clean work surface and cut each slice lengthwise in half to make 20 pieces of prosciutto in total. Wrap each shrimp with a slice of prosciutto, with the tail still hanging out. Thread the shrimp on a skewer and repeat the process until you have 4 skewers, each with 5 shrimp.

Now you're ready to cook the shrimp. Lightly coat a baking sheet with cooking spray, place the skewers on the sheet and place under the broiler. Broil for two minutes per side, remove the shrimp from the oven and serve at once with lemon wedges on the side.

Breakfast

Gluten Free Spinach Quiche

Number of servings: 6

Ingredients:

1 prebaked gluten free 9" pie crust (you can find these at health food stores)
1 cup prewashed baby spinach leaves, tightly packed
2/3 cup shredded Swiss or Jarlsberg cheese
3 large eggs
1 ¼ cups heavy cream
1 tsp salt
1 tsp black pepper
½ tsp nutmeg

Preparation:

Start by preheating your oven to 375 F. Whisk together the eggs, cream, nutmeg, black pepper and salt. Sprinkle half of the cheese on the bottom of the pie crust, followed by half of the spinach leaves. Pour about 2/3 of the egg mixture over the spinach, followed by the rest of the spinach and cheese, then the remaining eggs.

Bake for 30 minutes or until the quiche is set in the middle and golden brown on top. Remove from the oven and allow to rest for 5 – 10 minutes before slicing and serving.

Gluten Free Croissants

Number of servings: 12 croissants

Ingredients:

8 large eggs
2 cups of water
1 1/3 cup brown rice flour
1 cup of cold, unsalted butter
2/3 cup potato starch
2 tbsp sugar
1 tsp salt
cooking spray

Preparation:

Preheat your oven to 450 F and lightly coat a large baking sheet with cooking spray. Add the water and butter to a large saucepan and bring to a boil until the butter is melted. Whisk to combine and remove from heat.

Mix the dry ingredients in a large bowl and then add the water and shortening mixture. Stir until the dough pulls together into a ball. Allow the dough to cool for 10 – 15 minutes. Add the eggs one at a time, beating each egg into the dough until thoroughly combined. You should now have very sticky dough.

Spoon about 1/3 cup of dough onto the baking sheet for each croissant. Bake for 20 minutes. Reduce the heat to 350 F and bake for another 10 minutes. Remove from the oven, allow them to cool to room temperature and serve with the toppings of your choice. Individually wrap leftover croissants and refrigerate.

Pumpkin Muffins with Maple – Cream Cheese Filling

Number of servings: 12

Ingredients:

2 large eggs
1 cup brown rice flour
1 cup canned pumpkin
¾ cup sugar
½ cup canola oil
1/3 cup potato flour
¼ cup almond milk
4 tbsp tapioca starch
1 ½ tsp cinnamon
¾ tsp allspice
½ tsp ground ginger
½ tsp salt
1 tsp baking soda
¾ tsp xanthan gum (use corn starch if you can't find this)
½ tsp baking powder

The filling:

½ cup low fat cream cheese, softened at room
temperature

¼ cup powdered sugar
2 tbsp maple syrup

Preparation:

Start by preheating your oven to 350 F. Line cupcake or muffin tins with liners. Mix together all of the dry ingredients in a large bowl until well combined. Mix together the eggs and sugar in a separate bowl until smooth. Add the remainder of the wet ingredients and mix until smooth. Stir the dry ingredients slowly into the wet ingredients until well combined. Fill each muffin liner about ¾ full and set aside.

Now you can make the filling. Add the cream cheese, powdered sugar and maple syrup to a food processor and blend until very smooth. Spoon about 1 tbsp of the filling into each muffin liner. Bake for 25 minutes or until a toothpick inserted into the center of a muffin comes out dry or with just a few crumbs.

Remove the muffins from the oven and allow to cool in the tin for 5 – 10 minutes, then transfer the muffins to a cooling rack to cool to room temperature before serving.

Coconut Flour Pancakes

Number of servings: 6

Ingredients:

3 large eggs
3 tbsp coconut flour
3 tbsp coconut oil
3 tbsp coconut milk
1 tsp brown sugar
½ tsp baking soda
¼ tsp salt
a little canola oil, for cooking

Preparation:

In a medium sized bowl, whisk together the oil, eggs, coconut milk, salt and sugar. Mix in the remaining ingredients and add a little water until the batter reaches your desired consistency.

Heat a little canola oil in a frying pan or skillet. Pour in ¼ cup per pancake and cook until done on both sides. Serve hot with the toppings of your choice.

Turnip Hash

Number of servings: 4

Ingredients:

2 medium sized turnips, trimmed and grated
1 medium russet potato, grated
½ of a medium sized yellow or red onion, diced
1 tbsp olive oil
1 tbsp chopped Italian parsley
salt and black pepper, to taste

Preparation:

Mix together the shredded turnips and potatoes in a large bowl, then add the diced onion and a little salt and black pepper. Toss again to combine. Heat the olive oil in a large, heavy skillet over medium – high heat. Once the oil is hot, transfer the turnips and potatoes and cook for about 12 minutes, flipping over halfway through. Cook until crisp on both sides, sprinkle with chopped parsley and serve hot.

Crepes

Number of servings: 3 (2 crepes per serving)
1 large egg
2/3 cup whole milk
1/3 cup corn starch
2 tsp melted butter
a pinch of salt
a little canola oil, for cooking

Preparation:

Add all of the ingredients to a blender and mix until thoroughly combined. Drizzle a little bit of oil into a large, heavy skillet over medium high heat. Remove from heat and pour in about 2 tbsp of batter, swirling the skillet to spread the batter. Cook for about 30 seconds, or until the crepe browns around the edges and starts to pull away from the sides of the skillet. If the crepe doesn't brown, increase the heat slightly.

Lift the edge of the crepe gently with a spatula, grab with your fingers or tongs and flip over. Cook for another 20 seconds and transfer to a plate. Repeat the process until you've used up all of the batter. Enjoy with the sweet or savory fillings and toppings of your choice.

Berry Cornbread Muffins

Number of servings:

Ingredients:

1 large egg
1 cup fresh or frozen mixed berries, your choice
1 cup milk or almond milk
1 cup gluten free flour
¾ cup cornmeal
½ cup corn flour
¼ cup sugar
¼ cup canola oil
4 tsp baking powder
1 tsp vanilla extract
¼ tsp salt
zest of 1 lemon

Preparation:

Start by preheating your oven to 400 F. Line a 12 cup muffin tin with liners. Combine all of the dry ingredients in a large bowl and mix well to combine. Mix all of the wet ingredients until thoroughly combined in a separate bowl. Add the wet ingredients to the dry ingredients a little at a time, mixing until they're just combined. Fold in the berries gently. Divide the batter among the lined muffin cups, sprinkle with lemon zest and bake for 18 – 20 minutes, or until a toothpick inserted in the center of a muffin comes out clean. Allow to cool for at least five minutes, then transfer to a wire rack to cool to room temperature before serving.

Quinoa and Corn Cakes

Number of servings: 5 – 6 (10 – 12 cakes)

Ingredients:

1 cup cooked quinoa
1 large egg
2 scallions, trimmed and sliced thinly
½ cup water
½ cup vegetable broth
½ cup fresh or frozen corn (thaw first if using frozen corn)
1/3 cup diced red bell pepper
¼ cup shredded low fat mozzarella
¼ cup gluten free flour (your choice)
2 tbsp corn flour
2 tbsp milk or almond milk
½ tsp salt
½ tsp black pepper
a little canola oil, for frying
salsa, for serving (your choice)

Preparation:

Beat the egg in a medium sized bowl and then add the

remaining ingredients (except for the canola oil). Mix well to combine. If the batter is too wet, add another tbsp of flour. Heat a little canola oil in a large non-stick pan. When the oil is hot, add ¼ cup of the batter and press with a spatula. Cook as many at a time as you can while still leaving room between the cakes. Cook for about 3 minutes per side, or until golden brown. Serve immediately with the salsa of your choice.

Gluten Free Banana Bread

Number of servings: varies (1 8" x 4" loaf)

Ingredients:

1 ½ cups all purpose gluten free flour
3 medium ripe (or slightly overripe) bananas, mashed
2 large eggs
½ cup plain Greek yogurt
½ cup flax meal
½ cup unsalted butter, softened at room temperature
1 tbsp baking powder
2 tsp vanilla extract
½ tsp baking soda
½ tsp salt
¾ tsp each guar gum and xanthan gum (if your flour doesn't contain this already)
cooking spray

Preparation:

Preheat your oven to 375 F. Lightly coat a 8" x 4" loaf pan with cooking spray. Combine the dry ingredients in a large bowl with a whisk to combine. Cream the butter and sugar until fluffy in a separate bowl, then beat in the eggs until combined. Fold in the vanilla extract and yogurt. Add the dry ingredients to the butter mixture and beat until just combined. Add the mashed bananas and stir to combine. The batter should be thick and chunky.

Transfer the batter to your prepared loaf pan and smooth the top of the loaf with a spatula. Bake for 25 minutes, then tent the loaf pan with foil and continue baking for 1 hour, or until a toothpick inserted into the middle of the loaf comes out clean. Remove from the oven and allow to cool to room temperature before slicing and serving.

Buckwheat Pancakes

Number of servings: 12

Ingredients:

2 cups buckwheat flour
2 large eggs, beaten
1/3 cup powdered sugar
2 cups milk or almond milk
3 tbsp ricotta cheese
2 tbsp melted butter
1 tsp baking powder
a pinch of salt
a little oil, for cooking

Preparation:

Combine all of the ingredients in a mixing bowl and whisk together until smooth (but not totally smooth). Heat a little oil in a heavy skillet over medium heat. Once the oil is hot, add a little of the batter and cook until bubbles stop forming on the top. Flip and cook the other side until golden brown. Transfer to a plate and cover to keep warm. Repeat the process until the batter is used up. Serve hot with the toppings of your choice.

Desserts

Gluten Free Pecan Pie

Number of servings: 6 - 8

Ingredients:

The crust:
1 egg, lightly beaten
12 tbsp cold butter, cubed (1 ½ sticks of butter)
1 cup finely ground brown rice flour
½ cup arrowroot powder
½ cup amaranth flour
¼ cup white rice flour
1 tbsp brown sugar or turbinado sugar
1 tbsp very cold water
¼ tsp salt

Preparation:

Add the dry ingredients to a large mixing bowl and whisk to combine, then transfer to a food processor. Add the butter and pulse until the mixture takes on the texture of coarse crumbs. Add the egg and pulse until just incorporated. Add the water and pulse a few times to combine. If the dough doesn't hold together, add a little more water, ¼ tsp at a time until it can be formed into a ball.

Transfer the dough to a clean work surface lined with waxed paper. Flatten into a large disk. Wrap in wax paper and refrigerate for 1 – 2 hours before rolling out into a 10" circle between two sheets of waxed paper. Preheat your oven to 350 F. Carefully flip the dough into a 9" pie tin and press in to form a crust. Trim the edges and crimp with a fork. Pierce the crust in several places with a fork and bake for about 15 minutes or until golden brown. Remove from the oven and allow to cool while you make the filling.

The filling:
2 large eggs
1 cup pecans, plus extra pecan halves for topping the pie
2/3 cup sugar
½ cup light corn syrup
2 tbsp melted butter
1 tsp vanilla extract
½ tsp salt

Preparation:

Preheat your oven to 425 F. Add the eggs, corn syrup, butter, salt, vanilla extract and sugar to a food processor and pulse to combine. Add the pecans and pulse until the pecans are coarsely chopped. Pour the filling into the crust and top with pecan halves. Bake for 15 minutes, then reduce heat to 350 F and bake for another 30 minutes or until lightly browned. Remove from the oven and allow to cool on a wire rack before slicing and serving.

Gluten Free Chocolate Chip Cookies

Number of servings:

Ingredients:

3 cups almond flour
½ cup chocolate chips
½ cup butter, softened at room temperature
½ cup sugar
¼ cup chopped walnuts (this is optional, can be omitted if desired)
2 large eggs
2 tsp vanilla extract
½ tsp salt
½ tsp baking soda

Preparation:

Start by preheating your oven to 350 F. Cream the butter and sugar in a large bowl. Fold in the eggs and mix to combine. Add the baking soda, salt, almond flour and vanilla extract, then mix well. Fold in the chocolate chips and walnuts, if you're using them in this recipe. Scoop 1 tbsp of dough per cookie onto a foil lined baking sheet and bake for 12 – 14 minutes. Remove from the oven and allow to cool before serving.

Pumpkin Cake

Number of servings: varies

Ingredients:

The cake:
1 cup of canned pumpkin
3 large or extra large eggs
1 (15 ounce) package of gluten free yellow cake mix
½ cup of canola oil
¼ cup of turbinado sugar
3 tbsp of orange juice
1 tbsp of cinnamon
2 tsp of vanilla extract
¼ tsp of ground ginger
¼ tsp of ground cloves
cooking spray
The glaze:
1 cup of powdered sugar
2 tbsp orange juice

Preparation:

Start by preheating your oven to 350 F. Lightly coat a
bundt pan with cooking spray and dust with cinnamon;

shake out the excess. Add the yellow cake mix, canned pumpkin, sugar, orange juice, vanilla extract, eggs, ginger, remaining cinnamon and cloves to a large mixing bowl. Beat until well combined using an electric mixer or egg beater. Pour the batter into your prepared bundt pan.

Bake for 40 minutes and remove from the oven. Allow to cool for 10 – 15 minutes. Free the cake from the pan by running a thin, sharp knife around the edges of the cake. Invert the bundt pan over a wire rack and shake gently to remove the cake from the bundt pan. Allow the cake to cook completely on a wire rack (this will take at least 20 minutes). While the cake is cooling, you can make the glaze by whisking together the powdered sugar and orange juice in a small bowl. Spoon the glaze over the cake, slice and serve.

No-Bake Strawberry Pie

Number of servings: 6 – 8

Ingredients:

1 9" gluten free graham cracker pie crust
3 cups of strawberry yogurt
2 cups of sliced fresh strawberries
¾ cup of heavy cream
6 tbsp turbinado sugar
2 tsp of vanilla extract
½ tsp salt

Preparation:

Add the heavy cream, 3 tbsp of sugar and 1 tsp of vanilla extract to a mixing bowl and whisk until stiff peaks form in the mixture. Set aside. In a separate medium sized mixing bowl, add the strawberry yogurt, the other 3 tbsp of sugar, the other 1 tsp of vanilla extract and the salt. Stir until the sugar is dissolved.

Add the whipped cream and fold in to blend. Add the sliced strawberries and fold in. Transfer the mixture to the graham cracker crust and smooth the top of the pie with a spatula. Transfer the pie to the freezer and freeze until firm. Cover the pie with plastic wrap once completely frozen. When you're ready to serve the pie, remove it from the freezer and allow it to thaw for about 10 minutes before slicing and serving.

Pistachio Cheesecake

Number of servings: 6 - 8

Ingredients:

1 ¼ cups of gluten free flour
1 stick of unsalted butter
3 cups of milk
2 small packages of instant pistachio pudding
1 cup of cream cheese, softened at room temperature
1 cup of powdered sugar
1 cup of whipped topping (or make your own whipped cream)
½ cup of chopped pistachio nuts

Preparation:

The crust will take longer to make, so start by putting this together. Preheat your oven to 350 F. Melt the butter and blend with the gluten free flour and pecans in a food processor until it forms a crumbly dough like consistency. Spread the dough in a 9" x 13" baking dish and bake for 15 – 20 minutes, or until the crust becomes a light golden brown. Remove the crust from the oven and allow it to cool completely.

Now you can make the filling for your cheesecake. Mix together the softened cream cheese and the powdered sugar, then fold in half of the whipped topping or whipped cream. Spread the mixture on top of the crust once it has cooled to room temperature. Transfer to the refrigerator and chill for at least 30 minutes.

Next, mix the pistachio pudding mix with 3 cups of milk and beat for about 2 minutes or until it starts to thicken. Pour the pudding on top of the cooled crust and cream cheese filling. Return to the refrigerator and chill until the pudding has completely set. Top with the remaining whipped topping or whipped cream, slice and serve.

Brownies with Matcha

Number of servings: varies

Ingredients:

1 egg
½ cup of brown rice flour
¼ cup of white rice flour
¼ cup of tapioca flour
¼ cup butter
¼ cup (2 ounces) of unsweetened chocolate
¼ cup of dark chocolate chips
1/3 cup of turbinado sugar or sucanat
1/3 cup of coconut sugar
½ cup of coconut milk
3 tbsp of coconut milk
1 tsp baking powder
1 tsp vanilla extract
½ tsp salt
matcha powder*
cooking spray
* this is finely ground, powdered green tea. You can find matcha powder in Asian markets as well as in many larger grocery stores in the coffee and tea section.

Preparation:

Start by preheating your oven to 350 F. Melt the chocolate and butter in a double boiler over low heat. Once the chocolate and butter are melted, remove from heat and allow it to cool slightly. Lightly coat a 8" x 8" square pan with cooking spray and set aside.

Combine all of the dry ingredients in a large mixing bowl. Add the egg, vanilla extract and milk. Beat with an electric hand mixer or egg beater. When combined, add the chocolate and butter mixture. Beat at high speed until the batter is well mixed and creamy in texture.

Pour the batter into your prepared cake pan. Sprinkle the chocolate chips over the top of the brownies evenly and allow them to sink into the batter. Place the brownies in the oven and bake for 30 minutes, or until a toothpick inserted into the center comes out clean. Remove the brownies from the oven and allow them to cool in the pan. While the brownies are cooling, dust the top with matcha powder and cool to room temperature before slicing and serving.

Gluten Free Weight Loss Conclusion

The recipes in this book are meant to provide you with a good introduction to the gluten free lifestyle, whether your plan is to eliminate it from your diet for a shorter term weight loss or maintenance plan or to make a lifelong habit of eating a diet which does not contain this often problematic protein. By cooking these meals, you'll begin to get a feeling for how you can create meals without gluten and along the way, come up with some new gluten free recipes of your own.

As with any cookbook, you should feel free to experiment a little with the recipes. If you think a dish would benefit from a different herb, more or less garlic or so on, go right ahead – you're the chef here, after all. If you're less experienced in the kitchen, then you may want to follow these recipes as they are written until you gain a little confidence in your culinary skills, however.

Other than weight loss and better health, one of the biggest benefits of going on a diet like the gluten free diet is that it allows you to get a new perspective on cooking and can help you to become a more skilled and creative cook, which is never a bad thing. From appetizers to desserts, breakfast to dinner, there is almost nothing that you can't make gluten free; and of course, there are probably many foods which you already enjoy that contain no gluten – include these in your diet as well, provided that they follow the basic guideline of being as unprocessed as possible and of course, nutritious. Once you get gluten out of your life and learn how to live (and cook) without it, you may never go back again, even if you don't have a sensitivity to this common protein.

Section 2: Mediterranean Diet

Every solid weight loss plan requires increased attention on the foods you eat. But the contents of your diet, however healthy, cannot provide wellness if one fails to remember to structure their lifestyle accordingly. If you want to lose weight, finding solid information is the key to this step. That information can help you achieve the best mindset to reach your goals.

If the extremes of modern day fringe diets impose too great a demand upon your palate, it may perhaps be beneficial to look backwards in time for more natural and traditional diet based health solutions.

Whether your objective is to lose weight or eliminate a chronic health condition, more and more people nowadays are turning to the Mediterranean diet as a means to improve their overall wellness. Providing a delectable variety of proteins, vegetables, and favorite recipes dating back thousands of years, a Mediterranean diet is one, which can enable you a healthier lifestyle while still providing delicious meals.

It doesn't just taste delicious; it's good for you too. The

Mediterranean diet first came to the attention of the west in the mid 20th century when studies showed that people living in Southern Europe, where most recipes share much in common, not only had much longer life expectancy, but were comparatively free of chronic conditions such as heart attacks and hypertension compared to their northern neighbors.

It was perhaps a bit over-hyped a few decades ago when it was hailed, due to some misinterpreted facts in early studies, as a veritable fountain of longevity based on dietary factors alone. For example, at the time of the initial studies, the majority of Southern Europeans were still engaged in agricultural labor, and with private car ownership as well as public transport (in most areas) hard to come by, the people walked pretty much everywhere they went. Additionally, they didn't take notice of the more favorable work-life balance common in Mediterranean cultures, the early studies failed to report that an active lifestyle was part of the answer to why Southern Europeans lived longer, healthier lives. Despite this, it's a truism that no diet, however salubrious, is going to be of much benefit without an active lifestyle.

Before becoming the global sensation that it is today, the foodstuffs comprising the Mediterranean diet were based more on easy availability than on any profound ancient wisdom known by the region's early inhabitants, although human intervention played a significant role in which crops became dominant.

Unlike less favorable climates, with short growing seasons and a need for food that would last the long winters, both the choice and quantity of foodstuff in the Mediterranean was vastly greater than that found in less naturally blessed environments. Whereas the common people of the north subsisted mostly on bread, preserved meats, and a little cheese, inhabitants of the Mediterranean, with far more choices, naturally made a habit of eating a rich variety of foods.

As befits its namesake sea, the Mediterranean diet is very rich in seafood. The snaking coast lines and many islands meant that nearly all Southern Europeans had access to fresh fish, clams, mussels and calamari on a regular basis while most northerners only experience with seafood came in the form of salted cod from the distant Atlantic that had been marinating over a mule's back for 6 weeks in the summertime on its way inland. So can it really be surprising that most Germans grew to prefer sausage?

Long growing seasons meant that there was always

some freshly harvested produce in the local markets, so the inhabitants rarely had to resort to rat-infested stocks of grain like their climatologically challenged neighbors during sub-arctic winters.

History and trade had a hand in it too. Long before Roman times, the Mediterranean was a highway for the various peoples along its rim. Olives, Citrus fruits, grapes, as well as chickpeas and other legumes that comprise the heart of the Mediterranean diet were distributed via these early trade networks, and then mass-produced in industrial fashion on the vast Roman villas that dotted the body of water they, not unjustifiably, called *Mare Nostrum*, or "Our Sea".

Cash crops like Grapes, wool, and flaxseed were primarily exported, while cheap and easy to grow grains and vegetables were made available as the food supply of the armies of agricultural laborers and slaves upon whom the system rested. Obviously, it was in the Roman's interest for this vast labor force to be as well (yet cheaply) fed as possible. The 1000-year period of political and economic union forged by the Roman Empire did much to ensure that most ingredients composing the Mediterranean diet of today were eaten across the whole region thousands of years ago.

The typical Mediterranean diet is made up of over 30% fats. However, the saturated fat from red meat and heavy animal fats that lead to clogged arteries makes up only 8% of the total, due in large part to the relatively rare consumption of red meat and preference towards olive oil as a heating agent. Once again, geography plays a role. With most of the farmland along the Mediterranean crowded into fertile valley nestled between mountains or deserts, livestock was mostly used for dairy purposes. Indeed, before Southern European diets were influenced by modern habits, lamb was just about the only red meat consumed, and even then only sparingly, as wool was the main source of clothing.

This diet is not typical of all Mediterranean cuisine. In Northern Italy, for example, lard and butter are the usual heating agents for in cooking, and olive oil is used only for dressing salads and vegetables. In North Africa wine is religiously avoided by most of the locals.

Even though the diets of Southern European's themselves are steadily broadening, the health benefits of limiting your meal's ingredients to those traditionally found along the Med will provide long term benefits and provide a richness of flavor rarely found in the "fad" diets promoted by one weight loss guru or the next.

Key Ingredients and Recipes

As computer programmers like to say about code, "Garbage in, Garbage out", the same goes for the ingredients we put into our meals. The first step in using the Mediterranean diet to increase your health is to first learn of what it's composed of, and then using those ingredients in your daily meals.

Fruits and Vegetables

The Mediterranean region has volcanic soils and a 12-month growing season, so it is not surprising that the people of that area, on average, consume nine portions of fruits and vegetables every day. Mediterranean residents generally purchase their produce from farmers markets and produce stands. They also enjoy it when it's most flavorful by consuming "in season" produce.

Vegetables provide the most antioxidants needed for health and longevity when they are heated and processed only minimally. Even more important, the variety of vegetables and fruits commonly consumed gives people who have trouble sticking to diets a higher chance of success due to the greater choices available. In Addition to Mediterranean fruits and vegetables now consumed globally like oranges, grapes, and lemons, some of the key Mediterranean fruits and vegetables are:

Artichokes

Renowned for their flavor since ancient times, artichokes are in fact flower buds from a type of thistle plant. It is not advisable to eat artichokes raw, since only a small part of each bud is edible. In fact, prepping raw artichokes takes even an experienced chef a great deal of time. When cooked, however the tender bottoms on the inside of the bud's and the middle of the plant called the artichoke "heart" taste utterly divine. If you purchase raw artichokes (which are usually much cheaper due to the amount of effort it takes to prepare them for cooking), avoid those with leaves that point away from the middle of the plant center, because they will be mostly inedible fiber. If you wish to savor a traditional artichoke recipe, bake some with butter. Sprinkle some olive oil and vinegar over the finished artichokes and enjoy. Of course, if you want a quick snack, pre-cooked artichokes can be substituted. They are commonly available in cans or jars at most supermarkets.

Figs

A favorite across the entire Mediterranean region, the fig is a sweet fruit grown on the *Ficus carica* (fig tree). The Fig tree is a native to the Middle East but grows very well in the Mediterranean climate. Figs contain many antioxidants and are a good source of flavonoids and polyphenols. They are one of the highest plant sources of fiber and calcium, which promotes strong healthy bones.

Fresh figs do not have a very long shelf life. You will probably find dried figs or fig preserves more easily. If you are fortunate to find fresh figs try the ancient delicacy of dipping them in honey, or you might enjoy drizzling a little chocolate on them for a real burst of flavors.

Eggplants

Most Europeans know Eggplant as Aubergine. It is widely consumed cooked in savory dishes. Mistakenly it is referred to as a vegetable when if fact it is a fruit.

Eggplant is very popular in Mediterranean cuisine. The people of Lebanon and Israel grill the eggplant and then combine it with tahini, lemon juice, garlic and a bit of salt to make a dip called Baba Ganouj. It is served with warm pita. It is a key ingredient in Ratatouille, a vegetable relish with tomato, garlic, zucchini, onion and herbs from Southern France. And the delicious Greek Moussaka would just not be possible without eggplant.

Most Mediterranean eggplant has bitter juices that must be drained off before the eggplant is cooked. The best way to do this is simply sprinkle slices of eggplant with salt and let it sit for a while. The juices will be drawn off and the flesh will then be delicious.

Beans and Legumes

While many of the beans and legumes found in the Mediterranean diet were, like potatoes, brought from across the Atlantic during the 15th century, other has been a feature for thousands of Years. Black and red beans figure prominently in Spanish Cuisine. Fava Beans, Kidney beans, and lima beans as commonly featured in regional dishes as well. Chickpeas are featured prominently, being the basis of many stews in the Western Mediterranean, like Spanish *garbanzo* soup and in the east it is mixed with Tahini to produce delicious humus, a staple food, especially favored in the eastern

Mediterranean and the North African coast.

A Typical Mediterranean inspired salad could be made with leafy greens. Include some tomatoes, peppers, carrots, onions, beets and radishes and drizzle a little vinegar and olive oil on top. Make roasted vegetables like peppers and eggplant a regular addition to your diet. Gain maximum health benefits by striking meat from the menu two days a week. Meat is not the only source for protein. You can get plenty of good protein from beans and lentils.

Fish and Seafood

American grocery stores usually have tiny fish counters and enormous meat counters. This is right in line with the typical American diet that includes copious amounts of red meat and little seafood.

Seafood and fish should be more prominent in your diet. They are low in calories and high in omega-3 fatty acids.

Southern European diets, going all the way back to Julius Caesar's time, are high in mussels and clams, octopus, squid and other seafood. Of course most people of Southern Europe live within 20 miles of the sea. So they have ample access to these iron rich foods. Northerners on the other hand are land-based and subsequently have diets of more red meats. Simple logistics made this a reality since seafood could not be shipped to far without spoiling.

When selecting the method your seafood is prepared choose sautéed, grilled, steamed and roasted to keep the health benefits. Deep-frying in fat is obviously less healthy.

One example of a healthy alternative to frying would be to mix calamari in with pasta or rice. You could add saffron, mussels and some red peppers to the calamari and rice to make Spanish Paella.

Olive Oil

Saturated fats and hydrogenated oils should sound a loud "stay-clear" signal. A healthy Mediterranean Diet has no place for these two health thieves. The Mediterranean Diet gets some fat from fish and cheese but the majority is from olive oil. Olive Oil is very popular in the Mediterranean region. Grazing land is a premium and olive trees flourish. Each tree is capable of producing several gallons of oil per season. Olive oil is a wonderful dressing for salads, makes a good butter replacement on bread and offers many health benefits. It has been reported that olive oil can lower LDL (bad cholesterol) levels and is a good source of antioxidants. Both can reduce the risk of heart attack.

Garlic, Oregano, Basil, and Other Herbs

Many Mediterranean dishes include garlic, which is well known for its marvelous health benefits. Some benefits associated with garlic are:

- High in antioxidant compounds which promotes a healthy heart and immune system.
- Has germanium, which is an anti-cancer agent. Garlic has more germanium than any other herb.
- Lowers blood pressure, serum triglycerides, and LDL – cholesterol and prevents arteriosclerosis reducing the risk of heart attack and stroke.
- Improves joint health. Studies show garlic eaters were less likely to suffer osteoarthritis.
- You can increase your consumption of garlic by infusing it into the oils you cook with or adding some to the water you boil your pasta in.

For additional flavor boosts use spices like basil and oregano. You will add flavor to your food without increasing sodium in your diet.

Acetate, Borneol, Bisabolene, Carvacrol, Caryophyllene, Cymene, Geranyl, Linalool, Linalyl Acetate, Pinene, Terpinene and Thymol are all in the oils and leaves of Oregano and Basil, making both sources of internal and topical health benefits.

Basil is high in the essential mineral magnesium, which improves blood flow by relaxing blood vessels.

Many have found that eating basil regularly helps digestion. Studies have shown basil has strong antibacterial properties. These components battle parasites in the colon and intestines, as well as fight off some bacteria that are resistant to modern antibiotics.

Basil oil is a good remedy for stomach problems like indigestion, cramps and constipation. It is also effective at treating colds, flue and sinus infections. Studies show that it may help treat whooping cough, bronchitis and asthma.

With basils many health benefits you would do well always have some on hand. There really is no reason you can't, as it is one of the easiest herbs to grow. All you need is a sunny spot in the kitchen and a pot large enough to grow healthy roots.

Adding basil to your diet is easy, it is the primary ingredient in pesto sauce. For A tasty pesto sauce boil 2 parts spinach with 1 part basil add some ground pine nuts and olive oil and salt to taste.

Another way to add basil to your diet is to simply toss a few leaves into your favorite dish.

One more tip is to add basil oil to your salad dressing; the antibacterial components will fight bacteria on your vegetables and make them safer to eat.

Dry and fresh herbs add burst of flavor and amazing health benefits at the same time.

Whole Grains

When people think of the Mediterranean they think of bread, rice and pasta. Cheese and olive oil seasoned bread is a lunchtime staple. In Eastern Mediterranean regions flatbreads and pita are the standard. Wholegrain versions of these unleavened breads are heaped with nutritional value, all in a compact package.

If you are using the Mediterranean diet as for weight loss you should limit yourself to whole grain carbohydrates. You can add a bit of flavor with a little Baba Ghanouj, Hummus or simple Olive oil.

Pasta is by an large an Italian favorite, but it is very much acceptable in any Mediterranean diet as long as you are careful to avoid the savory northern Italian recipes which, with their heavy cream sauces, thick lathering of cheese, and use of fatty sausage or meatballs, are mainly designed to fortify a person against the bitterly cold winters in north Italy. Further south, pasta is typically served plain, with some seafood like mussels or clams, using garlic and olive oil or pesto sauce as extra flavor.

Just as importantly, bare in kind that much of Southern Europeans' health advantages stem from a relatively more relaxed and social-minded culture. In the United States, for example, people tend to eat rushed lunches, with a mere 30 minutes to move, eat, and hurry back. Often alone. Anyone seen partaking of an alcoholic drink in broad daylight may be frowned upon, even sneered at publicly, doing so in front of work colleges may even result in a long-winded speech from the boss. Southern Europeans will typically enjoy long lunch breaks, typically about 2 hours (In Spain, its followed by the *siesta,* during which the entire country essentially closes for business) with workmates, family or friends with a full bottle or two of drink lubricating the conversation. In short, they eat to ENJOY life rather than merely SUSTAIN it, and work is the MEANS of living rather than the REASON for it!

Cheese and Yogurt

As mentioned earlier, cows were too expensive to raise to be eaten frequently, so what cows there where traditionally employed producing dairy products. Yogurt was the most common, traditionally being easy to make, and lasting unrefrigerated much longer than fresh milk, a valuable feature during the hot summers. It was a common breakfast dish for the Romans, who commonly ate the plain variety with fresh fruits or honey as a flavoring.

Many Mediterranean cheeses such as feta and Brie are softer and less aged than northern counterparts. This is because, without a long, snowy winter, Southern Europeans had less need of food sources that would stay fresh for 4 months. Cheese and yogurt makes a very important nutritional contribution, which will become clear in the next section.

Protein Sources

As part of a well-balanced diet it is important to ingest sufficient levels of healthy protein. Cheeses that are eaten regularly in the Mediterranean diet including feta, mozzarella and goat cheese are all similar in that they contain a lot of protein in each portion. It is important to remember that protein is a crucial part of the growth process for muscle tissue. Since muscle requires much more energy than other cell types, developing more muscle will aid in speeding up your metabolism, intensifying your rate of weight loss. The seafood, beans and legumes described in a previous chapter are another excellent source **of low**-fat protein. Remember that meats like poultry, chicken, pork and Lamb are consumed, but in small portions only about 3 times a week. For example, chicken is traditionally included in rich dishes.

Key Nutritional Benefits of the Mediterranean Diet

Calcium and Magnesium

Residents of the Mediterranean coast consume yogurt and cheese on a regular basis. Both these foodstuffs are sources of the minerals calcium and magnesium. Calcium and magnesium are valuable to maintain healthy bones and are used by your brain and nervous system to transmit instructions throughout the body. Eating a diet rich in protein and healthy fats like the omega-3 in fish and the unsaturated type found in olive oil additionally increases your body's ability to absorb these and other beneficial vitamins and minerals. Followers of The Mediterranean diet ought to maintain a balanced intake of protein and fat, which makes the minerals, found within the cheese more effective.

"Good" Cholesterol Foods and Low Amounts of Saturated Fats

Even though high levels of it are considered quite harmful, Cholesterol is an essential part of the human body. It controls the flow of water and many other essential chemical compounds to each corner of your body. Cholesterol is a primary ingredient that your body transforms into essential hormones like estrogen and testosterone. Having enough of it in your liver allows you to properly process high-fat foods and helps you process vitamins A, D, and E. Including some of the low-fat cheeses favored in the Mediterranean diet will maximize your levels of good cholesterol while keeping the "bad cholesterol levels" low and within tolerable bounds. Many inhabitants of the Mediterranean shore favor cheese made from goat and sheep's milk. Goat and sheep cheese host less saturated fats and feature the primarily monounsaturated fats which promote a healthy heart.

Rich in Essential B Vitamins

Everyone knows that vitamins are important, but those numbered in the B complex group are additionally so. The ingredients of the Mediterranean diet provide a constant stream of B vitamins including niacin, thiamine, B-6 and B-12. These vitamins are the agents that transform the various proteins, fats, and carbs that end up in your belly into useful fuel to be used for developing muscles and energy. Foods featured in the Mediterranean diet such as Chickpeas, lentils, whole grains, and fish are all rich sources of b vitamins.

Healthy Mediterranean Habits

While considered a traditional, economically backwards region for the past few hundred years by their industrialized, rapidly growing northern neighbors, modernity eventually did arrive in countries of the Mediterranean coastline. However, while urban inhabitants have picked up their share of modern habits like driving and vegetating in front of the TV for extended periods, in the countryside and smaller towns, the people continue to live in a way that, in addition to the healthy diet, naturally promotes long and healthy lives. This is contributed to by both economic and cultural factors.

Healthy Mediterranean Habits 1: Get Some Sun

A high proportion of Southern European's still work in agriculture. It is not unusual to come across farms or vineyards that have been run by the same family for a dozen generations or more. The Mediterranean climate, with its hot dry summers and mild, wet winters, means that most regions can grow different crops year-round, so they don't have a 5 month winter break spent hiding from the cold and binge drinking like their northern neighbors do. This abundance of outdoor activity means they are out in the sun a lot, which means their skin produces a very high amount of vitamin D. Interestingly, skin cancer rates are lower among southern Europeans than people living in other sunny locations with similar climates, such as New Zealand. Some studies attribute this to the higher level of pollution in the upper atmosphere that filters out some of the UV radiation, while others attribute it to the fact that the inhabitants of the Mediterranean rim have had thousands of years to grow a genetic tolerance for sunlight.

Whichever is the case, there is no argument that a lot of time spent outdoors which gives your body the chance to produce its own vitamin D has great health benefits.

Healthy Mediterranean Habits 2: Walk wherever you can

Since Southern European towns and villages date *back* to the middle ages and beyond, they are compact and very pedestrian friendly. While many European Mediterranean residents' own cars, they still walk much more than Americans. This isn't just because the towns are smaller, traditionally, the center of social life in Mediterranean towns and villages revolved around the town square, known in various times and places as the agora (Greek), the forum, (Roman), the Plaza (Spanish) and the Piazza (Italian), the town center is where the cafes, local church, government offices, and daily outdoor markets are usually hosted. Even today on any evening, these venerable places swarm with young couples, families, and retired folks enjoying life together.

Mediterranean Habits 3: Social People are Happy, Healthy People

Social links are very strong on Mediterranean culture, commonly valued as much more important than their economic situation. Indeed, unlike the Anglo-Saxon obsession with measuring personal success with wealth, prestige, or position, Southern Europeans commonly measure their level of fulfillment by the quality of their family and social lives.

This is not just true in the countryside, where in the rugged valleys; the entire population is literally related to everyone else. While it is considered normal in certain countries to come home and catch up on work, it is more common along the Mediterranean to leave work and family completely separated (except, of course, in a family farm or business).

While family life is often the centerpiece of social life,

people typically "get on" with each other more. In the cafes and squares that dot the region, newly met strangers commonly swap stories and share drinks over a game like dominoes in Spain or lawn bowling in Italy.

The extra quality time with loved ones and friends spent on social and cultural pursuits is revealed through many studies to be an extra contributor to the lower incidences of anxiety, stress, depression, heart disease and depression among southern Europeans.

Even if you don't work on a farm, or it's impossible to do anything in your town without driving, incorporating a "Mediterranean Mindset" is a valuable addition to taking advantages of its cuisine. The extra exercise with keep you fit, and an extra focus on family activities will add incalculable value to your sense of personal fulfillment.

Medical Benefits

The Mediterranean diet food pyramid has little in common with the Western pattern diet. To Summarize, the top of the pyramid is red meat, which is consumed in small amounts a few times a month. Eggs, poultry and fish get served a few times each week. Small portions of yogurt and cheese are consumed regularly. Olives and olive oil are a regular accompaniment to each meal. Just above the Mediterranean diet's base is fruits and vegetables, with nuts and beans included. Pasta, bread, and other grains compose the bottom of the food pyramid. The Mediterranean diet overall is linked to a lower risk of heart disease and high cholesterol. This is due to the amount of healthy fat consumed from olive oil and cheese, and a more fulfilling cultural mindset in which family and social pleasure outranks work in the hierarchy of needs.

While several diets have been noted, the diet offering the strongest evidence of beneficial health effects to include reduced mortality is the Mediterranean diet.

Primarily a plant based diet; the Mediterranean diet has received many accolades for its high intake of dietary fiber and replacing saturated fats with healthy monounsaturated fats.

For decades westerners have been loath to salt and are surprised with the high salt content in the Mediterranean diet. Olives, anchovies, sardines, capers, salted fish roe, salt-cured cheeses are all staples in the Mediterranean diet, as are olive oil based salad dressings. Consider for a moment that our bodies rely on salt and need quite a bit every day. Studies confirm that Southern Europeans are not plagued with the heart problems that other Westerners suffer with. One main reason is that Southern Europeans are not exposed to the levels of saturated fats as Westerners since they consume much less red meat.

If you do switch your diet from the traditional Westerner fare to the healthier Mediterranean diet you would be well advised to limit your salt intake until your body balances out.

Of course diet is only one part of the health benefits of the Mediterranean culture. Add a balanced lifestyle of physical activity and outdoor labor and you complete the picture.

Genetics is a very small influence to the longer life spans

of the people of Southern Europe. Mediterranean
residents who changed their dietary habits and lifestyle
to mirror the less active and fat laden diet of Westerners
were found to have significantly increased their
incidence of heart disease.

There is considerable difference in incidence of heart
disease in the region between people who stick to
traditional foods and those who don't.

The comprehensive benefits of following the
Mediterranean diet in relation to good heart health is
essentially associative in nature; However they are
illustrated in the difference in the geographic frequency
of heart disease.

Medical research

While it was known that inhabitants of the Mediterranean enjoyed longer and healthier lives, there was little effort to quantify this until the mid 20th century. One of the first efforts to do so showed that males living on the Island of Crete had a low probability of suffering heart attacks, despite the fact that they ate a substantial amount of fatty foods. In common with other traditional Mediterranean diets, typical meals eaten here include a great deal of olive oil, bread, fresh fruit and vegetables, fish, dairy foods and wine.

Assuming that these low rates were not due to genetics, The Lyon Diet Heart Study included among its goals the aim of showing that any person eating foods found in the Cretan diet could see similar health benefits. The dietary change also required participants to eat much more vitamin C-rich fruit as well as whole-grain breads with a sharp reduction in red meat. Over the multi-year course of this study, the participant's death rate from all causes was reduced by a significant 70%! These results were considered so extraordinary that the supervisory committee decided to stop the study prematurely so that the results of the study could be made available to the public immediately.

This study proved that here were other benefits besides heart health to be enjoyed as a result of including Mediterranean ingredients in a diet plan, inspiring other research teams to quantify other health benefits. A 2008 study of the traditional Mediterranean diet found that if offers a great deal of protection against the development of type 2 diabetes. The study included more than 13 000 college aged students, who did not currently suffer from diabetes, whose eating habits were studied for a 10-year period.

After the ten year study had ended, researchers continued to track some of the participants. It was additionally revealed that who had subsequently continued to include Mediterranean ingredients in their diet had an 80% lower risk of diabetes

A more focused medical study revealed through a UK Medical institute in 2008 proved that persons whose diet is primarily composed of ingredients common in the Mediterranean diet lowered the odds of getting cancer and cardiovascular disease. The results reported a 9%, 9%, and 6% reduction in overall, cardiovascular, and cancer mortality respectively. Additionally a 13%

decrease in the odds developing of Parkinson and Alzheimer's diseases was shown as well.

A study published in the same Journal in 2009 shows that some aspects of the Mediterranean diet, including enhanced levels of vegetables without eating a lot of meat is more directly responsible for the overall low risk of mortality than other ingredients, like cereals, dairy, and fish.

Moderate alcohol intake, eating a substantial amount of fruits and nuts, are also associated with lower risk of an early death. Yet another research project published in February 2010 found that eating a mix of Mitterrand ingredients can aid in keeping the brain healthy by reducing the amount of micro strokes that play a large part in the development of senility.

Therefore, in addition to tasting great, offering many delicious ingredients to choose from, and promoting wellness, there is an abundance of scientific evidence proving the efficacy of the Mediterranean diet in reducing risk of a whole slew of chronic diseases. It should therefore be no surprise that the Mediterranean Diet is becoming a comprehensive popular and successful translational paradigm for the promotion of healthier lifestyles.

Extra Dieting and Wellness Tips

The family pet can be an ideal partner in any exercise routine you do alongside the Mediterranean diet. Pets provide unique weight loss motivation and help. You can walk, jog, or just play with your pet. Not only will you and your companion have fun, but also you will be helping yourself eliminate excess body fat from your body.

Instead of consuming sweet snacks every day, go with fruits. If you have been snacking on candy bars, chocolates and other unhealthy items, replacing them with fruits or healthy yet filling Mediterranean snacks like hummous and pita bread provides you with a healthier option with the benefits of the fruits' fiber, vitamins and minerals.

Fostering friendships with those who are fit and healthy can be beneficial to you. These people can serve as models for your desired weight goals. Also, you may be able to pick up extra tips and tricks on how to lose weight.

Make sure to maximize your water intake during the

day. If you drink about a half-gallon of water daily for a week and decrease your food intake, you are going to lose water weight. Avoid these strategies, improve your overall diet and increase your activity level for healthy weight loss.

Scan the outer perimeter of the grocery store for healthy foods. Fruits, vegetables, dairy items and meats listed later on in this guide. A little known grocery store fact is those foods in the center aisles tend to be prepackaged, preservative, salt, and sugar-laden and frequently lacking the essential nutrients for a healthy diet. By refraining from walking down these aisles, you will reduce the chance to purchase them.

Track all of the foods you eat and there amounts, as well as your daily activity levels. Studies show that those who keep a journal of these things eventually recognize certain patterns in their habits and find it easier to lose weight. Some people lose a lot more weight just because they pay attention more closely.

A great way to avoid snacking outside of set meal times is to suck on some ice when you're feeling the urge to snack or eat junk food. Sucking on an ice cube can help satisfy a desire to eat.

In order to shed pounds, you must realize the importance of a proper diet. Go through your kitchen and get rid of all the foods that would interfere with your weight loss, and replace them with traditional Mediterranean ingredients. Eating these healthy foods is the first thing that you have to do in shedding those extra pounds.

Try to avoid wearing lots of loose clothing when losing weight. It is common for overweight people to conceal their weight by wearing loose clothes. You should wear whatever you are comfortable in and not worry about concealing your shape. You are more likely to be cognizant of your weight if you wear clothing that is more form fitting.

Go to bed at a reasonable hour each night. A full eight hours of sleep is the ideal recommendation for adults. If you are thinking that staying up is helping you drop pounds, you are wrong. Getting enough sleep will keep your metabolism functioning properly.

Eating without focusing on portion sizes will lead to weight gain. If you aren't conscious of what you're eating at all times, you may end up consuming much more than you had intended to eat and that will harm your weight loss efforts. Be aware of how much you eat at every meal and you will likely eat less.

Consuming leftovers is a great way to maintain your weight loss regimen. Prepare enough extra portions at your healthy evening meal to take as your lunch the following day. You can make even more to get you through the whole week. This also helps you prepare a quick and simple meal without much fuss the following day.

Many times boredom and thirst can be misinterpreted as hunger pangs. Before you give in to a craving wait 15 minutes. During that 15 minutes drink some water and take a walk. If the hunger pangs persist then eat something.

Almost everyone enjoys the taste of French fries. They are the downfall of many a potential weight loser. Potatoes in general are not heavily featured in the Mediterranean diet, but when they are, they are more commonly heated via boiling or baking, rather than fried in artery-clogging grease. However, if you aren't quite able to quit French-fries altogether, take steps that help erase pounds instead of adding them, like baking them. Slice a small potato into fries, toss with a small amount of olive oil. Then season the slices with rosemary, salt and pepper and bake for thirty minutes in an oven set at

400 degrees. Loosen using a spatula and then bake for about 10 minutes longer. They are great with ketchup and have a much lower fat content, so you won't miss the deep-fried ones.

It is essential that you avoid food that triggers your appetite. This helps a lot of you are in control of your surroundings. You should avoid any contact with trigger foods in your home, your car or at work. If you are exposed to such items often, you may indulge even when not hungry.

Eat your largest meal of the day at lunchtime instead of at night. If you usually have a sandwich during lunch, try having it for dinner instead. You burn far more calories in the daytime and less in the evening, so it makes much more sense to consume more in the daytime and far less at night.

Keeping a healthy weight is the key to your future health. The way you live every day will decide if you can succeed in the long-term. Use what is available to you to make the changes in your life and to create a healthier body. Believe in yourself!

CPSIA information can be obtained at www.ICGtesting.com
Printed in the USA
LVOW07s1752090315

429814LV00029B/556/P

9 781631 879098